OUTLIVED

The Technique of Increasing Your Life by a Few More Years

Amanda M. Brooks

All rights reserved. No part of this publication may be reproduced, distributed, or transmitted in any form or by any means, including photocopying, recording, or other electronic or mechanical methods, without the prior written permission of the publisher, except in the case of brief quotations embodied in critical reviews and certain other noncommercial uses permitted by copyright law.

Copyright © (Amanda M. Brooks), (2023)

Table of Content

- Introduction..4
1. Unraveling the Mysteries of Alzheimer... 7
2. Exercise The Secret to Long-Lasting Vitality....................................... 38
3. Confronting and Preventing Cardiovascular Disease......................... 59
4. Innovative Approaches to Tackling the Menace of Cancer............................ 77
- Conclusion.. 104

Introduction

Certain facts loom large in the world of health and well-being. The most common cause of mortality in the US is heart disease, which casts a foreboding shadow. However, it is not unbeatable. The first step to empowerment is comprehending its subtleties. The armory of heart disease risk factors, both controllable and uncontrollable, provides insight into the battleground where prevention can change the outcome. In the struggle against this persistent foe, medications, state-of-the-art techniques, and lifestyle changes stand as powerful friends.

The tale of health, however, does not end there. The scope of vitality goes well beyond the confines of the heart. A powerful ally and protector against a different adversary cancer, emerges as physical activity. A startling truth revealed by recent studies is that nearly 46,000 cancer diagnoses could be avoided with just five hours of moderate-intensity exercise every week. In addition to providing hope and resilience, the power of movement—which includes everything from dancing to household chores—acts as a barrier against a variety of cancers.

The mind assumes center stage as we continue to navigate the maze of well-being. The mystery of cognitive function and its deep relationship to exercise is revealed. Physical activity and brain health have a strong relationship, which scientists have discovered during the past 20 years. Exercise stands out as a protector of cognitive toughness in the world of Alzheimer's disease, where an "increased oxidative state" imperils the mind's sanctuary. It improves memory, fosters neurogenesis, and cultivates brain plasticity, acting as a ray of hope against the onslaught of dementia.

The principles and advice in this book will serve as your compass as you navigate the confusing world of health. The skill of maintaining health and resilience will be discussed in these pages, not just as a lifetime dedication to the priceless gift of well-being but also as a means of coping with heart disease, cancer, and cognitive difficulties.

Chapter 1

Unraveling the Mysteries of Alzheimer.

Alzheimer's disease is a progressive form of dementia. A more general word for illnesses that impair memory, thinking, and behavior is dementia. The modifications impede day-to-day activities. Numerous factors, including diseases or brain damage, might contribute to dementia. The cause is occasionally a mystery.

60 to 80 percent of dementia cases, according to the Alzheimer's Association, are caused by Alzheimer's disease. Most patients with the condition are diagnosed after they turn 65. Alzheimer's disease that is diagnosed earlier is typically referred to as having a

"younger onset" or "early onset." Although there is no known cure for Alzheimer's, there are medications that can halt the disease's growth.

Statistical information about Alzheimer's

Even though many people have heard of Alzheimer's disease, it's still beneficial to be informed. These are some important specifics of this condition:

- Alzheimer's disease is a long-lasting, chronic disorder. It is an uncommon sign of aging.
- Dementia and Alzheimer's disease are distinct conditions. Dementia includes Alzheimer's disease.

- The degenerative nature of its actions on the brain results in a sluggish deterioration and gradual onset of symptoms.
- Although anybody can develop Alzheimer's disease, some people are more susceptible to it than others. The elderly and those with a family history of the ailment fall under this category.
- For those who have Alzheimer's, there is no one predicted prognosis. Some people have modest cognitive impairment for a long time, while others have symptoms that appear more suddenly and the disease progresses more quickly.

- Alzheimer's disease currently has no known cure, however, treatment can help reduce the illness's course and may enhance quality of life.
- Every person's Alzheimer's disease progresses differently.

How does Alzheimer's vary from other dementia types?

The distinctive abnormalities in the brain that distinguish Alzheimer's disease from other types of dementia may only be seen under a microscope during an autopsy. The following are frequently present in brains with Alzheimer's disease:

- Neurofibrillary tangles or fiber clusters within nerve cells
- Neuritic plaques are collections of nerve cells that are dying.

Reduced production of various brain chemicals, including acetylcholine, norepinephrine, serotonin, and somatostatin, which are essential for nerve cell communication, is another feature of Alzheimer's disease.

Causes of Alzheimer's

Even while age, one's health, one's family history, genetics, and aberrant protein deposits in the brain are thought to play a role in the disease's development, scientists still do not fully understand what causes it.

According to the National Institute on Aging, common causes include the following:

- Both age and ancestry
- A few genes
- Accumulation of abnormal proteins in the brain
- Environmental factors and additional risks
- Immune-system issues

Symptoms of Alzheimer's

Changes in short-term memory that can interfere with daily life, including forgetting words or names or how to go to a familiar location, are the first and most prevalent warning signs of Alzheimer's disease. Cooking or paying payments, for example, may become tough tasks.

The following are the most typical signs and symptoms of Alzheimer's disease, according to the Alzheimer's Association. However, every individual may experience symptoms differently. Possible signs include:

- Memory loss, especially short-term memory loss, that hampers work abilities
- Difficulty with routine activities
- Language issues Time and place disorientation
- Inadequate or lowered judgment

- Difficulties with abstraction
- Things becoming lost
- Alterations in behavior or mood
- Alterations in personality

When the illness reaches a severe level, a person may lose their capacity to recognize people, even those who are familiar to them, such as their child or spouse.

Alzheimer's illness diagnosis

Alzheimer's cannot be identified by a single test. Experts can diagnose Alzheimer's disease with roughly 95% accuracy and rule out other illnesses that may be similar. An autopsy is required to definitively identify the illness. Whether dementia is caused by a disease that may be treated must be determined by examination and evaluation. The following diagnostic techniques may be used to rule out Alzheimer's disease in addition to a thorough medical history and rigorous neurological, motor, and sensory examination:

- Challenge of the mind. This is a quick and easy test of memory and a few other typical cognitive abilities; it typically forms a component of a thorough neurological examination.
- Tests for the nervous system
- The drawing of blood
- (Spinal tap) Lumbar puncture. a treatment in which the lower back

(lumbar spine) is punctured with a hollow needle
- Urinalysis. Examination of urine in a lab for a variety of cells and substances, such as red blood cells, white blood cells, infections, or too much protein
- Imaging of the chest. a medical procedure that produces photographs of inside organs, bones, and tissues on film using imperceptible electromagnetic radiation beams
- A brain scan known as an EEG. a technique that uses electrodes placed on the scalp to continuously monitor the electrical activity of the brain

- CAT or CT scan stands for computed tomography scan. a diagnostic imaging process that creates axial or horizontal images (commonly termed slices) of the body using a combination of X-rays and computer technologies. The bones, muscles, fat, and organs are all visible in a CT scan, along with other bodily parts. General X-rays are less precise than CT scans.
- Imaging using magnetic resonance (MRI). a diagnostic method that creates detailed images of the body's organs and structures using a computer, radiofrequency technology, and massive magnets.

- A genetic test. It is possible to get some genetic testing, particularly in specific research settings. The decision to undergo genetic testing should be carefully considered, and discussion with a genetics expert is recommended because there is no known cure or effective treatment for Alzheimer's.

Medicine for Alzheimer's

Alzheimer's disease has no recognized cure. The progression of the disease can be stopped as much as possible by following your doctor's recommendations for drugs and other therapies.

Your doctor might recommend drugs like donepezil (Aricept) or rivastigmine (Exelon) for mild to early-stage Alzheimer's. High amounts of acetylcholine can be kept in your brain thanks to these medications. Your brain's nerve cells may be better able to transmit and receive information as a result. In turn, this might lessen some Alzheimer's signs and symptoms.

Only people with early-stage Alzheimer's disease should take the more recent medicine aducanumab (Aduhelm). It is believed to lessen the protein plaques that Alzheimer's disease causes to accumulate in the brain. However, other people wonder if the drug's potential advantages outweigh its risks.

Your doctor might recommend donepezil (Aricept) or memantine (Namenda) for the treatment of moderate-to-late-stage Alzheimer's. The effects of too much glutamate can be countered with memantine. When someone has Alzheimer's disease, their brain releases more glutamate, which harms brain cells.

To help treat Alzheimer's symptoms, your doctor may also prescribe antidepressants, anxiety medicines, or antipsychotics. These signs can include any of the following, depending on how the illness is progressing; Depression Problems, agitated hallucinations while sleeping. Although a person with Alzheimer's will need more care as time goes on, each person will uniquely experience the disease.

Additional Alzheimer's therapies

Changes in your way of life can help you manage your disease in addition to medicine. For instance, your doctor might devise the following methods to assist you or a loved one:

- Streamline chores
- Reduce misunderstanding
- Daily enough sleep, application of relaxing techniques
- Establish a soothing atmosphere

Your doctor and a team of healthcare professionals can help you maintain your quality of life at every stage of the Alzheimer's journey. A physical therapist can assist with staying active; a dietitian may aid with maintaining a healthy diet; and a pharmacist can assist with medication management.

Social workers, assist with locating resources and support respite care centers, provide short-term care for someone with Alzheimer's when their caregivers are temporarily unavailable at the hospice care center, manage symptoms in a peaceful and supportive environment at the end-of-life mental health professional, may work with the person with Alzheimer's as well as their caregivers

According to some research, vitamin E may be able to halt the progression of Alzheimer's disease, particularly when combined with drugs like donepezil that elevate acetylcholine levels in the brain. However, other studies revealed no advantages to vitamin E supplementation for Alzheimer's disease. Overall, additional proof is required.

Before taking vitamin E or any other supplements, be sure to see your doctor. Some of the drugs used to treat Alzheimer's disease may be affected by it. You can ask your doctor about several alternative and complementary therapies in addition to lifestyle changes.

How to stop Alzheimer's

There is no recognized treatment for Alzheimer's disease, just as there is no surefire way to avoid it. The best defense against cognitive aging we currently have is a healthy lifestyle. These actions could be helpful:

- Attempt to stop smoking. If you smoke, giving it up has immediate and long-term health benefits.
- Regularly moving around. Exercise reduces the risk of contracting a number of illnesses, such as diabetes and cardiovascular disease.
- Keep your thoughts active. Think about doing some cognitive training.

- Eat judiciously. Eat a fruit- and vegetable-rich, balanced diet to stay healthy.
- Maintain a socially active lifestyle. Your relationships with friends, your volunteer work, and your interests are likely to improve your general well-being. Before making any significant changes to your lifestyle, make sure to see your doctor.

The 7 Phases of Alzheimer

Common memory mistakes include losing your car keys, addressing your neighbor incorrectly, or forgetting to buy bread at the shop. But as we get older, forgetfulness becomes more common, and it's natural to start wondering what's normal, such as whether it's an indication of Alzheimer's disease. The most prevalent type of dementia, which is a word used to characterize the decline in cognitive function, is Alzheimer's disease. Alzheimer's disease can eventually make it difficult to do daily tasks like dressing and conducting conversations.

Knowing the symptoms of each stage of the disease can help you help someone you care about who is showing signs of Alzheimer's. Alzheimer's has no known cure, however, some drugs can temporarily stop the symptoms from becoming worse.

Keep in mind that everyone is affected by Alzheimer's differently. Each person's timing and intensity may vary, and it can be challenging to tell which stage your loved one is in because stages may overlap and are just intended as a general reference.

Stage 1: Before Symptoms

Alzheimer's-related alterations in the brain start before symptoms become apparent, much like with many other diseases. This period, which is frequently referred to as "pre-clinical Alzheimer's disease," probably starts 10 to 15 years before a person experiences symptoms. There is no treatment for this pre-clinical stage at the moment, but we anticipate developing drugs that will be able to stop the disease's progression before any symptoms appear.

As the risk of Alzheimer's disease rises with age, it's critical to maintain frequent primary care visits so that screening can identify the disease's early warning signals. Your loved one may be approaching the second stage of Alzheimer's if you observe that their cognitive abilities are starting to deteriorate.

Stage 2: Fundamental Forgetting

Everyone occasionally experiences forgetfulness, and as people become older, this is likely to happen more frequently. Alzheimer's disease's very early stages can resemble typical aging forgetfulness. Despite memory lapses, such as forgetting people's names or where they put their keys, your loved one can still drive, work, and interact with others. However, these forgetfulness lapses increase in frequency. As a result, you may be able to get them treatment earlier to delay the progression since you will likely notice this before your loved one does.

Stage 3: Prominent Memory Issues

The changes that many people may notice at this point will be harder to attribute to aging. This period is when most people receive their diagnosis because their daily routines are the most affected. Beyond simply forgetting names and losing things, this period is also characterized by common challenges. Your beloved might:

- Have problems recalling books or publications you've read recently
- Experience organizing and remembering plans are getting harder.
- Have more trouble remembering a word or name

Challenges at work or in social situations This stage may cause your loved one extra concern, and some people may even deny that anything is wrong. These emotions are natural, but waiting to see a doctor can only cause your problems to worsen. The best method to manage symptoms is to discuss care choices, including medication options, with your loved one's doctor.

Stage 4: Beyond Memory Loss

In this stage, brain injury frequently causes issues with language, organizing, and calculation skills, among other cognitive abilities besides memory. Your loved one may find it harder to complete daily duties as a result of these issues.

Your loved one will struggle with memory in great detail throughout this period, which can endure for many years. Significant facts about their lives, such as who they are married to or where they reside, may still be fresh in their memory. When compared to their recollection of current events, such as what they saw on the news or a conversation from earlier in the day, people tend to remember things from the distant past better.

At this moment, there are also the following difficulties:

- Uncertainty regarding the time and location of the day
- The risk of straying or getting lost is higher
- Alterations in sleeping habits, such as sleeping during the day and becoming agitated at night
- The challenge of selecting clothing that is appropriate for the climate or the situation

It's usual to feel depressed or withdrawn during this time, and circumstances that need a lot of thinking, like being in a social setting, can be quite frustrating. Your loved one might also go through additional personality changes as a result of brain cell destruction, such as feeling wary of other people, losing interest in activities, or feeling unhappy. Medications can frequently help these types of symptoms get better.

Stage 5: Lower Independence

It's possible that up until this point, your loved one had no real trouble surviving on their own. They were able to get by without your help most of the time, though occasionally you might have dropped by to see how they were doing.

At this point, likely, your loved one won't be able to recall significant others like their close friends and family. They could have a hard time picking up new skills, and even simple things like getting dressed might be too much for them. This period is also characterized by frequent emotional fluctuations, such as:

- Hallucinations: The perception of false objects
- Delusions: Untrue notions you mistakenly think are true
- The conviction that others are working against you

Stage 6: Severe symptoms

Being able to react to your surroundings, such as knowing what to do when the phone or fire alarm goes off, is a need when living alone. For those who have Alzheimer's, this gets challenging at stage 6. At this time, your loved one will be dealing with increasingly severe symptoms, making it harder for him or her to take care of themselves and making them more reliant on others.

Furthermore, at this phase, speaking may become challenging. Though they may still speak and use phrases, it can be difficult to get your loved one to express particular thoughts, like where they are in pain.

Increased anxiety, hallucinations, delusions, and paranoia are just a few of the significant personality changes that might keep happening. Your loved one can grow increasingly irritated with you as their level of independence continues to decline. You can discuss these situations with your care team and learn more about medications and behavioral techniques that may be helpful.

While not all patients will exhibit the aforementioned behavioral alterations, others may remain happy despite their illness. When they do happen, one should keep in mind that they are inexperienced at the time, therefore they shouldn't be held against you.

Stage 7: Lack of physical control

Brain cells are lost as a result of Alzheimer's disease, which over time may result in significant physical and mental disability. As their mind struggles to communicate and assign responsibilities properly, their body could start to shut down.

Your loved one will now have far more needs than before. To help them walk, sit down, and finally swallow, they might require 24-hour care. They may also be more susceptible to illnesses like pneumonia because of their decreased movement. Maintain good oral hygiene, apply an antibiotic ointment to cuts and scrapes right away, and make sure they have an annual flu shot to help prevent infections.

Chapter 2

Exercise The Secret to Long-Lasting Vitality

You desire to live longer. Be active. Exercise, as we all know, can help you stay in shape, lose weight, improve your balance, and reduce your risk of contracting several ailments, including heart disease. However several studies have indicated that exercise can lengthen your life.

This makes sense. After all, if exercise lowers your chances of developing cancer or heart disease, you've also decreased your likelihood of dying from these conditions. However, living longer has other benefits besides only lowering your risk of developing chronic diseases. Regular exercise keeps you youthful because it causes actual biological changes. Researchers at Brigham Young University discovered that those who were more active than those who were sedentary had longer telomeres, the end caps on chromosomes that shorten with age. This corresponded to a roughly 9-year difference in cell aging between active and inactive individuals.

Another study compared the heart, lungs, and muscles of 70-year-olds who were active, 70-year-olds who were sedentary, and 40-year-olds who were active. They discovered that the heart, lungs, and muscular strength of the active older men and women were equivalent to those who were 30 years younger.

One of the most crucial things you can do for your health is engage in regular physical activity. Being physically active benefits your bones and muscles, cognition, weight, illness risk, ability to carry out everyday duties, and ability to control your weight.

Adults will benefit in certain ways from sitting less and engaging in any amount of moderate-to-vigorous physical activity. One of the few lifestyle choices that has as much of an effect on your health as physical activity does is exercise.

A. Immediate Gains

Immediately following a session of moderate-to-vigorous physical activity, certain advantages of physical activity on brain health take place. Children aged 6 to 13 will experience enhanced thinking or cognition, while adults will see a decrease in the intensity of their momentary worry. Your thinking, learning, and judgment skills can stay sharp as you age with regular physical activity. It can also improve your sleep and lower your risk of anxiety and despair.

B. Management of Weight

The way you eat and how often you exercise are both very important for managing your weight. When you consume more calories through food and drink than you expend through exercise and other forms of physical activity, you acquire weight. Keeping your weight steady. Build up to 150 minutes a week of moderate physical exercise, such as dancing or yard work. With 30 minutes a day, five days a week, you might complete your 150-minute weekly target.

The amount of exercise that each person needs to manage their weight varies substantially. To reach or maintain a healthy weight, you might need to be more active than others.

For long-term weight loss: Unless you also change your eating habits and cut back on the number of calories you consume through food and drink, you will need to engage in a lot of physical activity. Regular exercise and a healthy diet are both necessary to reach and maintain a healthy weight.

C. Lower the Health Risk of Heart Disease

In the United States, heart disease and stroke are the two main causes of death. You can reduce your risk for these diseases by engaging in at least 150 minutes of moderate physical exercise each week. You can further reduce your risk by doing more exercise. You can lower your blood pressure and enhance your cholesterol levels by engaging in regular physical activity.

D. Metabolic syndrome and Type 2 Diabetes

Your risk of metabolic syndrome and type 2 diabetes can be lowered by engaging in regular physical activity. The metabolic syndrome is a condition marked by excess abdominal fat, high blood pressure, low HDL cholesterol, high triglycerides, and/or high blood sugar. Even if they don't get the recommended 150 minutes of moderate exercise each week, people can still benefit from exercise to some extent. Further physical exercise appears to lower the risk.

E. Maladies Infectious

Exercise has the potential to lower the risk of significant consequences from infectious diseases such as COVID-19, the flu, and pneumonia. For instance: COVID-19 is more likely to cause severe illness in those who engage in little to no physical exercise compared to those who do. CDC comprehensive analysis

A recent study demonstrates that, while inactivity increases the risk, physical activity is linked to a reduction in COVID-19 hospitalizations and deaths. Those who are more active may have a lower mortality rate from the flu or pneumonia. According to a CDC study, persons who follow the recommendations for aerobic and muscle-strengthening physical activity have a lower risk of dying from the flu and pneumonia than those who don't.

a few cancers

Your chance of developing a number of common malignancies is reduced by physical activity. Adults who engage in more physical activity are at lower risk of acquiring malignancies of the:

- Bladder
- Breast Colon (proximal and distal)
- Adenocarcinoma of the endometrium and esophagus
- Adenocarcinomas of the kidney, lungs, and stomach (cardia and non-cardia)

Regular physical activity helps cancer survivors improve their quality of life and physical health. It also helps them live longer.

F. Strengthen Your Muscles and Bones

Protecting your bones, joints, and muscles is crucial as you age because they support your body and facilitate movement. Maintaining strong bones, joints, and muscles can help you function better every day and participate in physical exercise.

You can build or maintain your muscle mass and strength by engaging in muscle-strengthening exercises like weightlifting. This is crucial for senior citizens who lose muscular mass and strength as they age. No matter your age, you can get even more benefits from muscle-building exercises by gradually increasing the weight and the number of repetitions.

G. Boost Your Daily Activity Capability and Avoid Falls

Daily activities include things like taking the stairs, shopping and playing with your grandchildren. Functional constraints are conditions that make it difficult for someone to carry out daily responsibilities. Middle-aged or older adults who are physically active are less prone to develop functional limitations.

A variety of physical activities improve physical function in older persons and reduce the incidence of falls and related injuries.

Include physical exercises like brisk walking, muscular building, and balance training. Multifaceted physical activity can be practiced as a part of a scheduled program at home or in a public space.

A fall can lead to a serious medical ailment called a hip fracture. If you're an older adult, breaking your hip might have drastic consequences. The risk of hip fracture is lower in physically active individuals than in inactive individuals.

H. Up the Chances of Living Longer

Increased moderate-to-vigorous physical exercise among US people aged 40 and older could avert an estimated 110,000 deaths annually. Even 10 minutes more every day could make a difference. Increasing the daily step count can lower the risk of premature death from any cause. The risk of premature death peaked at 8,000 to 10,000 steps per day for persons under the age of 60. The risk of early death for people aged 60 and over peaked between 6,000 and 8,000 steps per day.

I.   Manage recurring illnesses and disabilities

People can manage their chronic diseases and disabilities with regular physical activity. For individuals with arthritis, frequent exercise, for instance, can reduce pain and enhance quality of life while also enhancing function and mood. Aid type 2 diabetes patients in maintaining blood sugar levels while reducing their risk of heart disease and nerve damage.

There is never a wrong time to begin exercising.

You can still benefit from exercising even if you have been inactive for a long time. Studies have shown that adding modest physical activity to a person's daily routine can extend their life expectancy, even if they are overweight or have been inactive for a long time.

How much activity?

You can increase your longevity without training to be a top athlete. Regular, moderate exercise, such as brisk walking, has been shown to lengthen life expectancy by several years. For instance, those who engaged in at least 150 minutes of moderate exercise each week had a life expectancy improvement of around 7 years compared to those who did not. No matter one's weight, age, sex, or overall health, this benefit was observed.

Be sure to speak with your doctor if you haven't been active or are considering doing so. Your doctor could have suggestions for the kind and amount of activity you should start with based on your present state of health.

Mental Health And Exercise

Everyone is aware of how important exercise is for keeping one's body healthy. But did you know that regular exercise can also support mental wellness? According to research, those who frequently exercise have higher mental and emotional well-being, reduced rates of mental illness, and better physical health.

The likelihood of acquiring mental illness appears to be lowered by exercising. It also appears to be beneficial in the treatment of various mental health issues, such as anxiety and depression. For instance, evidence indicates that physical activity can be just as beneficial as antidepressants or psychological therapies like cognitive behavioral therapy for mild-moderate depression. Other therapy techniques can benefit from the combination of exercise.

Why can physical activity improve our mental health?

People who routinely exercise frequently do so merely because it makes them feel good. Your mood, focus, and alertness can all improve with exercise. Even a good attitude on life may result from it. The relationship between physical activity and mental health is nuanced. Mental disease, for instance, can both cause and result from inactivity. However, there are numerous ways that exercise might improve your mental health, including:

- When you exercise, the amounts of chemicals in the brain, including serotonin, stress hormones, and endorphins, vary.
- Sleeping better can be aided by regular exercise. A good night's sleep also aids with mood management.
- Your coping skills, sense of control, and self-esteem can all be improved via exercise. Regular exercisers frequently discuss how satisfying it feels to accomplish a goal.

- Exercise gives you the chance to try new things and might divert your attention from worrying thoughts.
- If you work with others, it provides an opportunity for social interaction and social support.
- You have more energy after working out.
- Your tensions may find a release through physical activity.
- By easing skeletal muscular tension, exercise might make you feel more at ease.

For those who suffer from mental illness, the physical advantages of exercise are crucial. Your cardiovascular health and general physical health both improve.

Asthma, heart disease, diabetes, arthritis, and other chronic physical illnesses are more common among those who struggle with their mental health, making this issue crucial.

Your mental health and exercise

You might be asking how much exercise you need to get to improve your mental health if regular exercise is not currently a part of your routine. The really good news is that working out doesn't need to be difficult or take a lot of time. According to studies, even light or moderate exercise can have a positive impact on your mood and thought processes.

According to Australia's physical activity and sedentary guidelines, adults should strive to engage in 2.5 to 5 hours of moderate physical activity per week, such as brisk walking or swimming. They also advise receiving 1.25 to 2.5 hours of strenuous exercise every week, such as jogging, quick cycling, or playing a team sport. You could also combine both vigorous and moderate activity.

Any exercise, though, is preferable to none. Exercises like stretching and yoga, as well as taking a stroll, can have a significant positive impact on your mind and body. Even simple housekeeping chores like cleaning, mopping, or vacuuming can provide a light workout.

Chapter 3

Confronting and Preventing Cardiovascular Disease

A group of illnesses known as cardiovascular disease (CVD) damages the heart or blood vessels (veins and arteries). Heart disease typically does not appear out of nowhere. It can be brought on by a confluence of socioeconomic, behavioral, and environmental risk factors, including high blood pressure, an unhealthy diet, high cholesterol, diabetes, obesity, smoking, renal disease, physical inactivity, dangerous alcohol use, and stress. High blood pressure, obesity, and diabetes are among other risk factors. The risk of cardiovascular disease can also be influenced by family history, ethnic background, sex, and age. The Cardiovascular Disease Prevention Program teaches participants how to change their behavior to ward against sickness, including what to eat for lunch and when to use the stairs instead of the elevator.

The Human Heart

The human heart is the body's hardest-working muscle, despite being only the size of a fist. Every time the heart beats, blood is pumped through the body, delivering nutrients and oxygen to every cell. The circulatory system, which consists of the heart, blood, and blood arteries, is made up of the heart, which is a muscular organ that pumps blood throughout the body. Through the blood vessels, the blood that is pumped provides nutrients and oxygen to the tissues and organs while also removing metabolic waste products like carbon dioxide.

The human heart is located in the middle of the chest, somewhat to the left of the center, between the lungs, and is about the size of a large fist. The heart beats approximately 100,000 times every day, pumping up to 7,500 liters of blood.

Why Do People Get Heart Disease?

The term "heart disease" refers to a group of illnesses and ailments that affect the circulatory system. There is a completely distinct reason for each type of heart disease.

Typical cardiac rhythms have a variety of causes, including

- Diabetic heart defects CAD
- Hypertension is an elevated blood pressure
- A few Medications
- Causes of a congenital cardiac condition

While a baby is still growing within the womb, this heart condition develops. Several significant heart conditions can be identified and treated early. Others might spend years without being diagnosed. With aging, your heart's structure may also change. This may result in a cardiac defect that could cause issues and difficulties.

Cardiomyopathy

Cardiomyopathy can take many different forms. Each category arises from a distinct circumstance:

- Dilated cardiomyopathy
- Cardiovascular hypertrophy
- Cardiomyopathy with restriction

Genetics, comorbidities, or other medical issues are some of the causes. Not every cause is completely understood.

Heart Disease Causes

Heart infections are most frequently caused by bacteria, parasites, and viruses. If uncontrolled infections in the body are not appropriately treated, they can potentially affect the heart. Depending on your situation, you may have different cardiovascular disease symptoms, such as:

- Chest discomfort, chest tightness, pressure, and pain
- Legs and/or arms ache and feel floppy or numb.
- Arms, neck, shoulder, jaw, and backache or pain
- Breathlessness Easily worn out through physical activity or exercise
- Rhythmic changes in your heart
- Chest palpitations or fluttering an extremely fast or slow heartbeat
- Fainting, feeling lightheaded, or dizzy
- weakness or weariness

- Swelling of the hands, legs, feet, ankles, or foot
- Fever
- Unusual patches or skin rashes
- Cough that is dry or ongoing

Intense chest discomfort, pain in the left arm or jaw, and breathing difficulties are all signs of a heart attack in males.

The same symptoms may occur in women, but they may have more widespread discomfort that affects their shoulders, neck, arms, belly, and back. Women could feel pain more like indigestion, and it might not be constant. It's possible that there isn't any pain, just unexplainable anxiousness, nausea, vertigo, palpitations, and cold sweats. Unexplained exhaustion can occur before heart attacks in women. In addition, compared to men, women usually experience fatal initial heart attacks that are more severe.

Seek emergency medical attention right away if you feel chest pain, difficulty breathing, or fainting. If you believe you may be having a heart attack, you should always dial the local emergency number. When cardiovascular disease, particularly heart disease, is discovered early, treatment is simpler. If you're worried about your heart health, talk to your doctor about the precautions you may take to lower your chance of developing heart disease, particularly if you have a family history of the condition.

Heart Disease Prevention

Up to 80% of heart attacks and strokes are avoidable, according to the World Health Organization. The majority of CVD-related deaths are caused by risk factors such as high blood pressure, high cholesterol, obesity, or diabetes. These conditions can, to a significant degree, be avoided or controlled by eating a balanced diet, engaging in regular exercise, and abstaining from tobacco. Monitoring your blood pressure, cholesterol, and blood sugar levels is also crucial.

1. Eat a balanced, healthy diet.

A healthy, balanced diet is essential to keeping your heart and circulatory system in good shape. A balanced diet should contain a mix of unprocessed and fresh foods, such as enough fruit and vegetables (at least five pieces daily), whole grains, nuts, and meals low in saturated fats, sugars, and salt. Avoid processed foods, which frequently have high salt content, and hydrate yourself frequently.

2. Regular exercise

Your health can be improved and maintained with just 30 minutes of moderate-intensity exercise five days a week. Adults (18–65) and seniors (65+) should strive to engage in 150 minutes or more per week of moderate-intensity physical activity or 75 minutes or more per week of high-intensity activity. Every day, kids and teenagers should engage in 60 minutes of physical activity that ranges from moderate to vigorous.

Try to incorporate exercise into your daily routine by taking the stairs rather than the elevator or getting off the bus a few stops sooner and walking the remaining distance. Exercise is a fantastic strategy to reduce stress and maintain a healthy weight, both of which are risk factors for cardiovascular disease.

3. Keep a healthy body weight

Reduce your intake of calories from fats and carbohydrates, increase your intake of fruit, vegetables, whole grains, and nuts, and engage in regular exercise to lower your chance of being overweight or obese. You can keep a healthy body weight by exercising for at least 60 minutes most days of the week.

4. Avoid using tobacco

Your risk of coronary heart disease will be cut in half within a year after quitting and will gradually return to normal if you do so. Avoid areas where there is a lot of smoke because doing so greatly raises your risk of having a heart attack. No level of cigarette exposure is safe; all kinds of tobacco are toxic. Talk to your doctor about creating a personalized plan if you're having problems quitting tobacco.

5. Avoid beverages

Alcohol use has no safe level, and its harmful effects outweigh any putative protective advantages by a wide margin. While drinking less may lower your risk of CVD, research suggests that abstaining from alcohol altogether is best for your health. When individuals stop drinking alcohol, even moderate drinkers experience improved health.

6. Control stress

Stress can tighten the arteries, increasing the risk of heart disease, particularly in women. You may regulate your stress levels by exercising, taking deep breaths, relaxing your muscles, and making time for the things you enjoy. Don't be hesitant to talk to someone or ask for help if you feel like things are getting out of hand.

7. Remember your numbers

Knowing your numbers is crucial for maintaining heart health. To assess and manage your risk of developing cardiovascular disease, it is crucial to regularly check your blood pressure, cholesterol, and blood sugar levels.

- Be aware of your blood pressure: Hypertension, often known as high blood pressure, is one of the main risk factors for heart attacks and strokes. It's crucial to get it periodically examined and, if necessary, to take the necessary steps to lower it, which may include dietary modifications, greater physical activity, and medication. It typically has no symptoms.

- Understand your cholesterol: Blood cholesterol levels that are too high put you at risk for cardiovascular problems like heart attacks and strokes. Normal blood cholesterol levels can be maintained with a balanced diet and, if necessary, the use of the proper drugs.
- Know your blood sugar levels: If your doctor advises it, you should follow the essential precautions to control your blood sugar. Diabetes, or having high

blood sugar, increases your risk of heart attacks and strokes.

8. Take your medicine as recommended.

You might need to take medicine if you have a higher risk of having heart disease or stroke. Statins to control blood cholesterol, low-dose aspirin to avoid blood clots, insulin for diabetes, and blood pressure-lowering pills are a few examples of these. Make sure you follow your regimen and take the medication that your doctor has prescribed.

What are a few heart disease risk factors?

Heart disease has numerous risk factors. Some are under our control, while others are not. Approximately 47% of Americans have at least one risk factor for heart disease, according to the CDC. Among these dangerous elements is excessive blood pressure. High-density lipoprotein (HDL), or "good" cholesterol, levels are low and cholesterol is high.

One risk factor that is under your control is smoking. According to the National Institute of Diabetes and Digestive and Kidney Diseases, people who smoke have a twofold increased risk of having heart disease.

Because high blood glucose levels raise the risk of heart attack (CAD), people with diabetes may also have an increased risk of heart disease. Keeping your blood sugar under control if you have diabetes can reduce your risk of heart disease. People who have both diabetes and high blood pressure are more likely to develop cardiovascular disease.

Risk factors outside of your control

The following are other heart disease risk factors: family history, ethnicity, sex, and age. Even while you can't manage these risk factors, you might be able to keep an eye on how they're affecting you.

A male relative under the age of 55 who has a history of CAD is particularly worrisome than a female relative who is younger than 65.

Chapter 4

Innovative Approaches to Tackling the Menace of Cancer

The development of new cancer treatments to decrease the side effects of current ones has been a major focus of several research efforts over the past 10 years. The main cause of mortality worldwide is cancer. As cancer progresses, tumors become extremely heterogeneous, resulting in a mixed population of cells with a variety of molecular characteristics and therapeutic responses. This variability, which is crucial to the establishment of resistance phenotypes encouraged by selective pressure upon treatment delivery, can be observed both at the geographical and temporal levels.

Typically, cancer is handled as a single, uniform disease, and tumors are viewed as a whole cell population. Therefore, to develop accurate and effective medicines, a thorough knowledge of these complicated events is crucial.

To administer traditional chemotherapeutic medications in vivo, increase their bioavailability and concentration around cancer tissues, and enhance their release profile, nanomedicine provides a flexible platform of biocompatible and biodegradable technologies. Various procedures, including therapy and medical diagnosis, can make use of nanoparticles.

Extracellular vesicles (EVs), which have a role in the development of cancer, the alteration of the microenvironment, and the progression of metastatic illness, have gained a lot of attention recently as efficient drug delivery vehicles. Due to their anti-proliferative and pro-apoptotic qualities, natural antioxidants and several phytochemicals have lately been offered as anti-cancer adjuvant therapy. The intracellular organelles or tumor vasculature are just two examples of the target areas of targeted therapy, which spares the surrounding tissue. As a result, the specificity of the treatment is greatly enhanced while its drawbacks are diminished.

Another alternative is based on gene therapy and the creation of tumor suppressors and apoptosis-inducing genes, or the targeted silencing mediated by siRNAs, which is currently being studied in several clinical studies throughout the world. Thermal ablation of tumors and magnetic hyperthermia are opening up new opportunities for precision medicine by enabling the localization of treatment in incredibly small and precise regions. Alternatives to more invasive procedures like surgery may be possible using these methods.

Additionally, emerging disciplines like radiomics and pathomics are assisting in the creation of creative methods for gathering massive amounts of data, developing novel therapeutic approaches, and accurately predicting patient responses, clinical outcomes, and cancer recurrence. With their combined efforts, these strategies will be able to provide cancer patients with the most tailored treatments, demonstrating the need to combine many professions to produce the best outcomes.

The Technology Transforming Cancer Research and Treatment

Thanks to some technical advancements that have resulted in advancements in the ways we identify, visualize, comprehend, and treat cancer, what previously appeared unattainable in the field of cancer research is now a reality. Exploring and employing these technologies further may pave the way for accelerating the fight against this illness.

CRISPR, artificial intelligence, telemedicine, the Infinium Assay, cryo-electron microscopy, and robotic surgery are just a few of the technologies and advances that are accelerating the fight against cancer. CRISPR scientists never dreamed of having the ability to rapidly and simply alter the genetic makeup of living cells. But because of CRISPR, which functions like a pair of scissors and can accurately remove, insert, or modify particular sections of DNA inside cells, that is now feasible. A side study conducted out of curiosity on how bacteria defend themselves against viruses led to the discovery of this revolutionary gene-editing method. In 2020, Drs. Jennifer Doudna and

Emmanuelle Charpentier received the Nobel Prize for their key CRISPR research. More studies are looking into CRISPR-made cancer medicines, and the first US clinical study of CRISPR-made cancer immunotherapy started a year earlier. Trials to employ CRISPR inside the human body are also starting. Although CRISPR is a game-changer, there are still limitations to the technology and ongoing debates over the ethics of gene editing. CRISPR, however, is a powerful technology that has the potential to dramatically progress not only cancer research but also other sectors.

A. Machine Intelligence

What if doctors could utilize a computer simulation to construct a virtual version of you, a "digital twin," so they could "explore" treatments and project potential results before offering you individualized treatment options? Thanks to developments in artificial intelligence (AI), it is no longer science fiction. Teaching a machine to reason, act, and acquire knowledge is the goal of artificial intelligence. Large volumes of data can be easily analyzed with this technique, which is very useful in scientific study. AI is being used by the National Cancer Institute (NCI), the Department of Energy, the Frederick National Laboratory for Cancer Research, and a transdisciplinary team of researchers to advance the creation of digital twins for cancer patients. Others use it to customize radiation dosages for patients by analyzing imaging data and electronic health records. Even population-based cancer data is being quickly analyzed with AI to calculate the likelihood of certain malignancies. And these are just the very beginning in terms of how AI might alter the way cancer care is delivered.

B. Telehealth

Even in a pandemic, clinical trials and cancer care delivery are essential. To provide cancer patients with treatment and care remotely, many healthcare organizations taking part in the NCI Community Oncology

Research Program (NCORP) have effectively expanded or adopted telehealth methods. These hospitals and clinics are utilizing telehealth for remote health monitoring, video visits, and even in-home chemotherapy to increase safety and convenience for both patients and providers across the nation. Additionally, telehealth facilitates access to cancer treatment and clinical trials for a wider range of patient populations over a larger geographic area. You might have utilized telehealth procedures outside of cancer treatment and contributed to almost one-third of medical appointments that were conducted virtually last year. Even if it is becoming more and more common, not all care can be given remotely. There are difficulties in ensuring the equitable use of remote healthcare technologies, but researchers are attempting to solve them.

C. Cryo-EM

You may believe that the newest iPhone has a fantastic camera, but you may not be familiar with cryo-electron microscopy (cryo-EM).Cryo-EM, which has resolutions so high they were unheard of just a decade ago, can take pictures of molecules that are ten thousandths the breadth of a human hair. Researchers rebuild 3-D images of molecules that enable scientists to investigate how they behave by analyzing hundreds of thousands of cryo-EM images for quality, similar to how people filter through numerous candid photos before sharing the "good" ones on social media. This entails a greater comprehension of how cancer cells develop, endure, and interact with treatments and other cells. Recent research using cryo-EM revealed the interactions between a treatment for chronic myeloid leukemia and ribosomes, a molecular machine inside cells, and produced the most complete picture of a human ribosome ever. This breakthrough might aid in the creation of cancer and other disease treatments.

D. Infinium Assay

What can genotyping, a tool for reading and comparing genetic information across individuals, tell us about cancer? The Illumina-developed Infinium Assay, which is employed by businesses like 23andMe and Ancestry, is a procedure and a collection of tools that examines millions of single nucleotide polymorphisms, or SNPs, the most prevalent kind of genetic variation. SNPs can be used to identify cancer-causing genes and shed light on the formation, progression, and risk of the disease. The test, which was developed with assistance from NCI's Small Business Innovation Research program, was at first viewed with suspicion regarding whether this technology was technically feasible. It is a convincing example of innovation that was supported by tax dollars. The assay is now utilized for a variety of purposes, including cancer research, ancestry reports, the NIH's All of Us Research Program, and even genetic studies of plants to determine the elements that influence their resistance to insects and drought.

E. Automated Surgery

Robotic surgery can facilitate a quicker recovery and return to normal life. Patients who need to have their prostate gland removed, because they have prostate cancer, can now have treatments that historically required cutting a large incision from the navel to the pubic bone performed using robotic arms that enter the body through microscopic incisions. Using a specialized console, the surgeon can control the arms while seeing a magnified view of the surgical site in real-time. In the case of prostatectomy, a patient could leave the hospital as soon as the day after surgery thanks to robotic surgery's reduced blood loss and pain. In a circumstance where a few millimeters could represent the difference between eradicating all malignant tissue and potentially injuring healthy tissue, the robotic arms' delicate, precise movements might make all the difference.

Avoiding Cancer

Between 30 and 50 percent of cancer cases can be avoided. The most economical long-term approach to cancer control is prevention. In addition to ensuring that people are given the knowledge and assistance, they need to adopt healthy lifestyles, WHO works with Member States to develop national policies and programs aimed at increasing exposure to and decreasing awareness of cancer risk factors.

The WHO Global Action Plan for the Prevention and Control of Noncommunicable Diseases 2013-2020 offers a road plan to reduce premature mortality from NCDs by 2025 by focusing on many of the risk factors listed below:

1. Tobacco

There are more than 7000 compounds in tobacco smoke, at least 250 of which are known to be dangerous, and at least 69 of which are known to cause cancer. More than 8 million people worldwide die from cancer and other diseases each year as a result of tobacco use, which is the single biggest preventable risk factor for cancer mortality. Around 80% of the 1.1 billion smokers worldwide reside in developing and middle-income nations.

2. Alcohol

According to the International Agency for Research on Cancer, alcohol is a Group 1 carcinogen that is toxic, psychoactive, and addictive and is causally associated with 7 different cancers, including oesophageal, liver, colorectal, and breast cancers. Each year, there are 740,000 new cancer cases linked to alcohol intake. Alcohol use is a contributing factor in one in twenty cases of breast cancer worldwide.

Light to moderate alcohol use was linked to about 23,000 new cancer cases in the EU in 2017, accounting for 13.3% of all cancers linked to alcohol and 2.3% of all cases of the 7 cancer categories related to alcohol. About 11,000 of these cancer cases, or about half, were breast cancers in women. Additionally, about 8500 of the cancer patients linked to light to moderate drinking (or more than a third) had a light drinking level.

Alcohol consumption increases the chance of developing a variety of cancers, including those of the breast, liver, pharynx, larynx, esophagus, and oral cavity. The amount of alcohol consumed correlates with an increased risk of cancer. 400,000 deaths globally, mostly in men, were thought to be caused by alcohol-related malignancies in 2016.

3. Infections

In low- and middle-income nations, cancer-causing diseases including hepatitis and the human papillomavirus (HPV) account for up to 25% of cancer cases. Vaccines against the hepatitis B virus and specific types of HPV can reduce the risk of acquiring cervical and liver cancer, respectively.

environmental damage

According to estimates, outdoor air pollution caused 4.2 million premature deaths worldwide in 2016, with lung cancer deaths accounting for 6% of all premature fatalities. Additionally, household air pollution from cooking with solid fuels and kerosene causes up to 4 million individuals to pass away early from illnesses.

4. Workplace carcinogens

It is commonly known that bladder cancer, mesothelioma, and lung cancer are all directly caused by occupational carcinogens. For instance, asbestos exposure at work is largely to blame for mesothelioma, a cancer of the outer lining of the lung or chest cavity.

5. Radiation

All forms of ionizing radiation exposure raise the chance of developing a variety of malignancies, including leukemia and other solid tumors. Younger ages at which exposure occurs and higher exposure levels both raise the risks. Basal cell carcinoma (BCC), squamous cell carcinoma (SCC), and melanoma are the three main kinds of skin cancer that are brought on by ultraviolet (UV) radiation, particularly solar radiation. Effective preventive strategies include avoiding excessive exposure, applying sunscreen, and wearing protective gear. Due to its link to ocular and skin melanoma malignancies, UV-emitting tanning systems are now also categorized as human carcinogens.

6. Increasing knowledge and awareness

The uptake of services and the number of dropouts in the cancer care cascade will increase with improved provider and patient understanding. It is crucial to educate front-line medical staff on how to accurately describe risk factors, identify cancer symptoms and signs, and quickly send patients who require medical attention.

Following a nationwide awareness campaign, the percentage of patients in Malaysia who presented with late-stage breast cancer decreased from 77 to 37 percent. The employment of cancer survivors as ambassadors is one of the tactics being tested in China to raise breast cancer awareness and early diagnosis. The basic healthcare workforce in Panama is undergoing standardized training, and the country is increasing the use of needle biopsies for diagnosis.

7. Enhancing Established Initiatives And Removing Obstructions

In some nations, cutting-edge care delivery approaches that make use of platforms for communicable diseases are being successfully implemented. For instance, Botswana has a long history of successfully integrating cryotherapy and the "see and treat" cervical cancer screening method into its effective HIV/AIDS program, with the help of numerous partners, including the World Bank. Similar to this, in Kenya, with funding from the World Bank and the Access Accelerated project, a chronic illness model based on an HIV/AIDS platform emphasizes early case discovery, linking to treatment, and task shifting to enhance the detection and management of cervical and breast cancer.

To help governments analyze and better manage bottlenecks in cancer control efforts, numerous diagnostic analyses have been created. In Brazil, a World Bank research highlighted ongoing problems with cancer treatment, including substantial access inequities, a breakdown in the continuity of care, and late-stage diagnosis (38 percent of cases were stage III/IV).

Due to a lack of equipment, treatment options, or gaps in accurately recording cases in the cancer registries, women in Ukraine were still lost at various stages of the screening, diagnostic, and treatment cascade, according to an analysis carried out in two provinces with assistance from the World Bank.

8. Assisting Those With Cancer

It will be crucial to empower and inspire cancer patients, their families, and members of civil society organizations to join forces in the fight against cancer. During their cancer journey, survivors can be knowledgeable advocates for others, sharing stories and assisting them in better coping with the condition. In many nations, cancer associations and civil society support groups have proven to be effective advocates and a sounding board for cancer patients and their families.

The patient's point of view has a significant impact on all of us and serves as a reminder of the many obstacles they confront as well as the opportunity to increase their chances of survival. A soon-to-be-released report funded by the World Bank chronicles the patient's journey from the patient's point of view in Kenya. We in the global health community must collaborate with the public and corporate sectors as well as civil society to advance early cancer detection, increase access to high-quality care, and ensure financial security against this potentially bankrupting condition.

Elizabeth, a 38-year-old mother of two from the eastern Kenyan county of Meru, had the good fortune to receive cervical cancer treatment and is currently in remission. Despite the hardships she faced, her struggle with cancer came to a more encouraging conclusion. Patients who overcome the odds and battle this fatal illness are more needed than ever.

Conclusion

Heart disease, cancer, and the close link between exercise and cognitive health have all been explored in detail. As we get to the end of this illuminating journey, we are not only left with knowledge but also with a clear call to action—to embrace the art of living a full life.

The vulnerability of heart disease, which is frequently seen as an impossible task, has been exposed. We may arm ourselves against this mighty foe by using information as our shield and lifestyle adjustments as our sword. Despite the promise provided by medications and surgical procedures, it is our daily decisions that ultimately determine our fate.

As a protector against cancer's unrelenting march, physical activity, formerly a faraway goal, is now recognized. Moving serves as our defense against this foe, and a mere five hours of weekly dedication might pave the road for a healthier future.

Exercise and cognitive vitality work together to promote resilience in the mental sphere. Physical activity helps the brain's incredible capacity for adaptation, which increases life expectancy and ensures that people have vivid memories and intellectual acuity throughout their lifetimes.

Keep in mind that this book is a spark for change as we draw to a close. These pages' lessons and advice can be used as a starting point for living a life that goes beyond the ordinary. Savour the gift of time, take care of your health and embrace the adventure. You discover the secret to living a meaningful, long life by doing this.

Printed in Great Britain
by Amazon